MIDNIGHT LIGHTS PUBLISHING HOUSE

PRESENTS:

WORLD'S BEST MOTHER

EAT FOR TWO

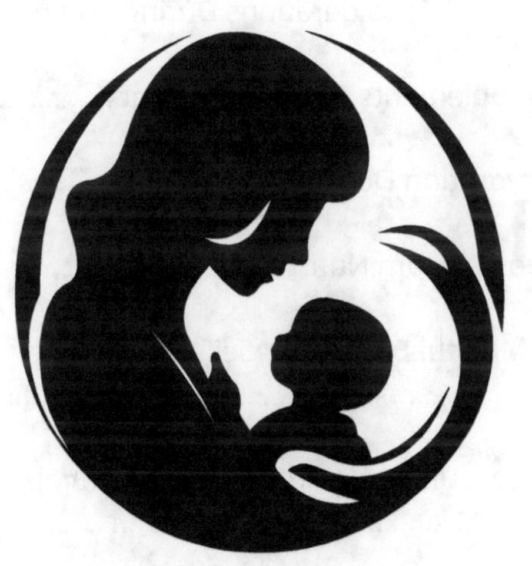

AUTHOR OF THE BOOK:

RACHEL GUARDIAN

TABLE OF CONTENTS

Chapter 1: Nutrient Requirements During Pregnancy

Introduction to Nutrient Requirements

During pregnancy, the body undergoes significant changes to support the growth and development of the fetus. Adequate nutrition is essential during this time to ensure the health and well-being of both the mother and the baby. In this chapter, we will explore the specific nutrients that are crucial for a healthy pregnancy and discuss why they are important for maternal and fetal health.

Folic Acid

Folic acid, also known as folate, is a B vitamin that plays a critical role in fetal development, particularly in the early stages of pregnancy. It is essential for the formation of the neural tube, which later develops into the baby's brain and spinal cord. Adequate folic acid intake can help prevent neural tube defects such as spina bifida and anencephaly.

Additionally, folic acid is involved in DNA synthesis and repair, making it important for cell division and growth. Pregnant women need increased levels of folic acid to support the rapid cell growth occurring in the developing fetus.

Iron

Iron is another vital nutrient during pregnancy, as the body requires more iron to support the increased blood volume and to supply oxygen to the growing fetus. Iron deficiency during pregnancy can lead to anemia, which can increase the risk of preterm birth and low birth weight.

Iron is also essential for the baby's brain development and overall growth. Pregnant women need to consume more iron-rich foods or iron supplements to meet their increased needs during pregnancy.

Calcium

Calcium plays a crucial role in the development of the baby's bones, teeth, muscles, and nerves. During pregnancy, the demand for calcium increases to support the growth and mineralization of the fetal skeleton. If the mother's calcium intake is insufficient, the baby will draw calcium from her bones, which may increase the risk of osteoporosis later in life.

In addition to bone health, calcium is also important for muscle function and blood clotting. Pregnant women should ensure they consume an adequate amount of calcium-rich foods such as dairy products, leafy greens, and fortified foods.

Omega-3 Fatty Acids

Omega-3 fatty acids, particularly docosahexaenoic acid (DHA) and eicosapentaenoic acid (EPA), are essential for the development of the baby's brain and eyes. These fatty acids are critical components of cell membranes and are involved in neurological and visual development during pregnancy and infancy.

Pregnant women should aim to include sources of omega-3 fatty acids in their diet, such as fatty fish (e.g., salmon, sardines), flaxseeds, chia seeds, and walnuts. Omega-3 supplements may also be recommended for those who do not consume enough from dietary sources.

Vitamin D

Vitamin D plays a vital role in calcium absorption and bone health, making it essential during pregnancy for both the mother and the baby. Adequate vitamin D intake helps ensure proper skeletal development in the fetus and reduces the risk of conditions such as rickets and osteomalacia.

In addition to bone health, vitamin D may also play a role in immune function and may help reduce the risk of certain pregnancy complications, such as preeclampsia and gestational diabetes.

In the following sections of this chapter, we will delve deeper into each of these nutrients, discussing their specific functions, recommended intake levels during pregnancy, dietary sources, and potential supplementation when necessary. It is important for pregnant women to be aware of their nutrient requirements and to make informed choices to support the health and development of their baby.

Folic Acid

Folic acid, also known as folate, is a B vitamin that plays a critical role in fetal development, particularly in the early stages of pregnancy. It is essential for the formation of the neural tube, which later develops into the baby's brain and spinal cord. Adequate folic acid intake can help prevent neural tube defects such as spina bifida and anencephaly.

Importance for Maternal Health:

- **Prevention of Neural Tube Defects:**
  Folic acid supplementation before and
  during early pregnancy is crucial for
  reducing the risk of neural tube defects,
  which are serious birth defects affecting
  the brain, spine, or spinal cord.
- **Supports DNA Synthesis:** Folic acid is
  involved in DNA synthesis and repair,
  making it important for cell division and
  growth. Pregnant women need
  increased levels of folic acid to support
  the rapid cell growth occurring in the
  developing fetus.

Importance for Fetal Health:

- **Neural Tube Development:** Folic acid
  is essential for the proper closure of the
  neural tube, which occurs during the first
  few weeks of pregnancy. Adequate folic
  acid intake at this stage is critical for
  preventing neural tube defects.
- **Brain and Nervous System
  Development:** In addition to neural tube
  closure, folic acid plays a role in the
  development of the baby's brain and
  nervous system. Sufficient folic acid
  levels during pregnancy support healthy
  neurological development in the fetus.

Sources of Folic Acid:

- **Fortified Foods:** Many grain products, such as bread, cereal, pasta, and rice, are fortified with folic acid in many countries as a public health measure to help ensure adequate intake, particularly among women of childbearing age.
- **Leafy Greens:** Dark, leafy green vegetables such as spinach, kale, and collard greens are natural sources of folate.
- **Citrus Fruits:** Citrus fruits like oranges and grapefruits contain moderate amounts of folate.
- **Legumes:** Beans, lentils, and peas are good sources of folate.

Recommended Intake:

- **Preconception:** Women of childbearing age are advised to consume 400 to 800 micrograms (mcg) of folic acid daily, ideally from a combination of foods and supplements, to reduce the risk of neural tube defects in case of unplanned pregnancy.
- **During Pregnancy:** Pregnant women should aim for 600 mcg of folic acid per day to support fetal development. Some women may require higher doses under the guidance of their healthcare provider, especially if they have certain risk factors for neural tube defects.

Supplementation: Folic acid supplements are commonly recommended for women planning pregnancy or during the early stages of pregnancy to ensure adequate intake, as it can be challenging to obtain sufficient amounts from diet alone.

Conclusion: Folic acid is a crucial nutrient for both maternal and fetal health during pregnancy. Ensuring adequate intake through a combination of dietary sources and supplementation can help reduce the risk of neural tube defects and support healthy fetal development. Pregnant women should consult with their healthcare provider to determine the appropriate folic acid intake for their individual needs.

Iron

Iron is another vital nutrient during pregnancy, as the body requires more iron to support the increased blood volume and to supply oxygen to the growing fetus.

Importance for Maternal Health:

- **Prevention of Anemia:** Iron deficiency during pregnancy can lead to anemia, a condition characterized by a low red blood cell count or hemoglobin levels. Anemia can cause fatigue, weakness, dizziness, and other symptoms that can impact maternal health and well-being.

- **Supports Oxygen Transport:** Iron is a component of hemoglobin, a protein in red blood cells that carries oxygen from the lungs to the rest of the body. During pregnancy, the body needs more iron to produce additional red blood cells and support the increased oxygen demands of the mother and the growing fetus.

Importance for Fetal Health:

- **Fetal Growth and Development:** Adequate iron intake during pregnancy is essential for supporting fetal growth and development. Iron is necessary for the baby's cells to grow and divide, and it plays a role in the formation of hemoglobin in the fetal blood.
- **Reducing Risk of Preterm Birth and Low Birth Weight:** Iron deficiency anemia during pregnancy is associated with an increased risk of preterm birth and low birth weight, which can have long-term consequences for the health and development of the baby.

Sources of Iron:

- **Lean Meats:** Beef, pork, and poultry are excellent sources of heme iron, which is more easily absorbed by the body compared to non-heme iron found in plant-based foods.

- **Seafood:** Certain types of seafood, such as shrimp, oysters, and clams, are rich in iron.
- **Beans and Lentils:** Legumes such as lentils, chickpeas, and kidney beans are good sources of non-heme iron.
- **Dark Leafy Greens:** Spinach, kale, and Swiss chard are rich in iron and other nutrients.
- **Fortified Foods:** Fortified cereals, bread, and pasta can provide additional iron.

Recommended Intake:

- **Preconception:** Women of childbearing age are advised to consume 18 milligrams (mg) of iron per day to meet their nutritional needs and prevent iron deficiency.
- **During Pregnancy:** Pregnant women should aim for 27 mg of iron per day to support the increased demands of pregnancy and prevent iron deficiency anemia. Some women may require higher doses under the guidance of their healthcare provider, especially if they have risk factors for iron deficiency.

Supplementation: Iron supplements are commonly recommended for pregnant women, especially those who are at risk of iron deficiency or who have difficulty meeting their iron needs through diet alone. However, supplementation should be taken under the guidance of a healthcare provider to avoid excessive intake, which can lead to gastrointestinal side effects.

Conclusion: Iron is essential for both maternal and fetal health during pregnancy. Ensuring an adequate intake of iron-rich foods and, if necessary, iron supplements can help prevent iron deficiency anemia and support healthy pregnancy outcomes. Pregnant women should discuss their iron needs with their healthcare provider and follow their recommendations for supplementation if needed.

Calcium

Calcium plays a crucial role in the development of the baby's bones, teeth, muscles, and nerves. During pregnancy, the demand for calcium increases to support the growth and mineralization of the fetal skeleton. If the mother's calcium intake is insufficient, the baby will draw calcium from her bones, which may increase the risk of osteoporosis later in life.

Importance for Maternal Health:

- **Bone Health:** Pregnancy can lead to a temporary loss of bone density in some women as the fetus draws calcium from the mother's bones to support its own growth. Adequate calcium intake during pregnancy helps maintain maternal bone health and reduces the risk of osteoporosis later in life.
- **Muscle and Nerve Function:** Calcium is essential for muscle contraction, nerve transmission, and the release of hormones and enzymes. Maintaining adequate calcium levels during pregnancy supports overall maternal health and well-being.

Importance for Fetal Health:

- **Bone and Tooth Development:** Calcium is a primary building block for the baby's bones and teeth. Adequate calcium intake during pregnancy ensures that the fetal skeleton develops properly and reduces the risk of skeletal abnormalities.
- **Muscle Function:** Calcium is involved in muscle contraction and nerve signaling in the fetus, supporting proper movement and development in utero.

Sources of Calcium:

- **Dairy Products:** Milk, cheese, yogurt, and other dairy products are excellent sources of calcium. Opt for low-fat or fat-free options to reduce saturated fat intake.
- **Leafy Greens:** Dark, leafy green vegetables such as kale, collard greens, and broccoli are rich in calcium.
- **Fortified Foods:** Some foods, such as fortified orange juice, tofu, and breakfast cereals, are fortified with calcium to help individuals meet their nutritional needs.
- **Fish with Edible Bones:** Canned fish with soft, edible bones, such as canned salmon or sardines, are good sources of calcium.
- **Nuts and Seeds:** Almonds, sesame seeds, and chia seeds are nutritious snacks that provide calcium.

Recommended Intake:

- **Preconception:** Women of childbearing age are advised to consume 1,000 milligrams (mg) of calcium per day to meet their nutritional needs and support bone health.
- **During Pregnancy:** Pregnant women should aim for 1,000 to 1,300 mg of calcium per day to support the increased demands of pregnancy and fetal development. The exact recommendation may vary based on individual factors and maternal age.

Supplementation: In some cases, healthcare providers may recommend calcium supplements for pregnant women who are unable to meet their calcium needs through diet alone or who have risk factors for calcium deficiency. However, it's important to consult with a healthcare provider before starting any supplementation regimen during pregnancy.

Conclusion: Calcium is essential for both maternal and fetal health during pregnancy. Ensuring an adequate intake of calcium-rich foods and, if necessary, calcium supplements can help support bone health, fetal development, and overall pregnancy outcomes. Pregnant women should discuss their calcium needs with their healthcare provider and follow their recommendations for supplementation if needed.

Omega-3 Fatty Acids

Omega-3 fatty acids, particularly docosahexaenoic acid (DHA) and eicosapentaenoic acid (EPA), are essential for the development of the baby's brain and eyes. These fatty acids are critical components of cell membranes and are involved in neurological and visual development during pregnancy and infancy.

Importance for Maternal Health:

- **Heart Health:** Omega-3 fatty acids have been shown to support heart health by reducing inflammation, lowering triglyceride levels, and promoting healthy blood pressure.
- **Mood Regulation:** Some studies suggest that omega-3 fatty acids may play a role in mood regulation and may help reduce the risk of perinatal depression in pregnant and postpartum women.

Importance for Fetal Health:

- **Brain Development:** DHA, in particular, is a major structural component of the brain and retina. Adequate intake of omega-3 fatty acids during pregnancy supports the growth and development of the baby's brain, nervous system, and visual pathways.
- **Eye Development:** Omega-3 fatty acids are also important for the development of the baby's eyes and vision. DHA is found in high concentrations in the retina, where it plays a crucial role in visual function.

Sources of Omega-3 Fatty Acids:

- **Fatty Fish:** Fatty fish such as salmon, mackerel, sardines, and trout are excellent sources of EPA and DHA.

- **Fish Oil Supplements:** Omega-3 fish oil supplements are available in capsule or liquid form and can provide a concentrated source of EPA and DHA. It's important to choose high-quality supplements that are free from contaminants such as mercury.
- **Plant-Based Sources:** Certain plant foods, such as flaxseeds, chia seeds, hemp seeds, and walnuts, contain alpha-linolenic acid (ALA), a precursor to EPA and DHA. However, the conversion of ALA to EPA and DHA in the body is inefficient, so plant-based sources may not provide as much of these omega-3 fatty acids as fish sources.
- **Fortified Foods:** Some foods, such as eggs, yogurt, and milk, may be fortified with omega-3 fatty acids to enhance their nutritional content.

Recommended Intake:

- **Preconception:** Women of childbearing age are encouraged to consume omega-3 fatty acids as part of a healthy diet to support overall health and well-being.
- **During Pregnancy:** Pregnant women should aim to consume at least 200 to 300 milligrams (mg) of DHA per day to support fetal brain and eye development. This can typically be

achieved through a combination of dietary sources and, if needed, supplementation.

Supplementation: Pregnant women who do not consume enough omega-3 fatty acids through diet alone may consider taking a fish oil supplement containing EPA and DHA under the guidance of their healthcare provider. However, it's important to choose supplements that are specifically formulated for pregnancy and are free from contaminants.

Conclusion: Omega-3 fatty acids are essential for both maternal and fetal health during pregnancy. Consuming adequate amounts of omega-3-rich foods or supplements can support fetal brain and eye development, as well as maternal heart health and mood regulation. Pregnant women should aim to include omega-3 fatty acids as part of a balanced diet and consult with their healthcare provider if considering supplementation.

Vitamin D

Vitamin D plays a vital role in calcium absorption and bone health, making it essential during pregnancy for both the mother and the baby. Adequate vitamin D intake helps ensure proper skeletal development in the fetus and reduces the risk of conditions such as rickets and osteomalacia.

Importance for Maternal Health:

- **Bone Health:** Vitamin D is necessary for the absorption of calcium from the intestines and the regulation of calcium levels in the blood. Maintaining adequate vitamin D levels during pregnancy supports maternal bone health and reduces the risk of osteoporosis and fractures later in life.
- **Immune Function:** Some research suggests that vitamin D may play a role in immune function and may help reduce the risk of certain infections and autoimmune diseases.

Importance for Fetal Health:

- **Skeletal Development:** Vitamin D is essential for the development and mineralization of the fetal skeleton. Adequate vitamin D intake during pregnancy supports the growth and strength of the baby's bones and teeth.
- **Reducing Risk of Rickets:** Severe vitamin D deficiency during pregnancy can lead to rickets, a condition characterized by soft, weak bones and skeletal deformities in the baby. Ensuring sufficient vitamin D intake helps prevent this condition.

Sources of Vitamin D:

- **Sunlight:** The primary source of vitamin D is sunlight exposure, as the skin synthesizes vitamin D when exposed to ultraviolet B (UVB) radiation from the sun. Spending time outdoors during peak sunlight hours without sunscreen can help increase vitamin D production.
- **Fatty Fish:** Fatty fish such as salmon, mackerel, and tuna are good dietary sources of vitamin D.
- **Fortified Foods:** Some foods, such as fortified milk, orange juice, yogurt, and breakfast cereals, are fortified with vitamin D to help individuals meet their nutritional needs.
- **Egg Yolks:** Egg yolks contain small amounts of vitamin D, although the concentration may vary depending on the hen's diet and exposure to sunlight.

Recommended Intake:

- **Preconception:** Women of childbearing age are advised to consume 600 international units (IU) of vitamin D per day to support overall health and well-being.
- **During Pregnancy:** Pregnant women should aim for 600 IU of vitamin D per day to meet their increased needs during pregnancy. Some women may require higher doses under the guidance of their healthcare provider, especially if

they have limited sun exposure or other risk factors for vitamin D deficiency.

Supplementation: In some cases, healthcare providers may recommend vitamin D supplements for pregnant women who are unable to meet their needs through diet and sunlight exposure alone. However, supplementation should be taken under the guidance of a healthcare provider to ensure appropriate dosage and safety.

Conclusion: Vitamin D is essential for both maternal and fetal health during pregnancy. Ensuring adequate intake through diet, sunlight exposure, and, if necessary, supplementation supports maternal bone health, fetal skeletal development, and overall pregnancy outcomes. Pregnant women should discuss their vitamin D needs with their healthcare provider and follow their recommendations for supplementation if needed.

Chapter 2: Healthy Eating Guidelines During Pregnancy

Introduction to Healthy Eating During Pregnancy

Maintaining a balanced and nutritious diet is crucial during pregnancy to support the health and well-being of both the mother and the baby. In this chapter, we will provide practical advice on how to achieve a balanced diet during pregnancy, including information on portion sizes, food groups to focus on, and tips for incorporating a variety of nutrient-rich foods into meals and snacks.

Importance of a Balanced Diet

A balanced diet during pregnancy provides essential nutrients that support fetal growth and development, help prevent pregnancy complications, and promote maternal health. By consuming a variety of nutrient-rich foods from different food groups, pregnant women can ensure they are meeting their increased nutritional needs and supporting optimal pregnancy outcomes.

Food Groups to Focus On

- **Fruits and Vegetables:** Aim to include a variety of colorful fruits and vegetables in your diet to provide essential vitamins, minerals, and antioxidants. Choose fresh, frozen, or canned options, and aim to fill half of your plate with fruits and vegetables at each meal.
- **Whole Grains:** Choose whole grains such as brown rice, quinoa, whole

wheat bread, and oatmeal for their fiber, vitamins, and minerals. Incorporate whole grains into meals and snacks to provide sustained energy and support digestive health.

- **Protein-Rich Foods:** Include lean sources of protein in your diet, such as poultry, fish, eggs, tofu, legumes, and nuts. Protein is essential for fetal growth and development, as well as maternal tissue repair and hormone production.
- **Dairy or Dairy Alternatives:** Consume dairy products or fortified dairy alternatives such as almond milk or soy milk to ensure an adequate intake of calcium and vitamin D. Choose low-fat or fat-free options to reduce saturated fat intake.

Portion Sizes and Meal Planning

- **Balanced Meals:** Aim to create balanced meals that include a combination of carbohydrates, protein, and healthy fats. Use portion control to ensure you're not overeating, and listen to your body's hunger and fullness cues.
- **Snack Smart:** Choose nutrient-rich snacks such as fruits, vegetables with hummus, Greek yogurt, or whole grain crackers with cheese. Snacking between meals can help maintain energy levels and prevent overeating at mealtime.

- **Hydration:** Drink plenty of water throughout the day to stay hydrated, especially as pregnancy increases fluid needs. Limit intake of sugary beverages and caffeinated drinks, and aim to consume most of your fluids from water.

Tips for Incorporating Variety

- **Experiment with New Foods:** Try new fruits, vegetables, grains, and protein sources to keep meals interesting and diverse.
- **Meal Prep:** Plan and prepare meals in advance to ensure you have nutritious options readily available. Batch cooking and freezing meals can save time and make healthy eating more convenient.
- **Food Safety:** Practice proper food safety techniques, such as washing fruits and vegetables, cooking meat thoroughly, and avoiding unpasteurized dairy products and raw seafood, to reduce the risk of foodborne illness.

Conclusion: Maintaining a balanced diet during pregnancy is essential for supporting maternal and fetal health. By focusing on nutrient-rich foods, practicing portion control, and incorporating a variety of foods into meals and snacks, pregnant women can ensure they are meeting their increased nutritional needs and promoting optimal pregnancy outcomes. Consult with a healthcare provider or registered dietitian for personalized nutrition advice and guidance throughout pregnancy.

Chapter 3: Foods to Include and Avoid During Pregnancy

Introduction to Food Choices During Pregnancy

Making informed food choices is crucial during pregnancy to ensure the health and well-being of both the mother and the baby. In this chapter, we will provide guidance on foods to include in a healthy pregnancy diet, as well as those to limit or avoid due to potential risks.

Foods to Include for a Healthy Pregnancy

- **Fruits and Vegetables:** Incorporate a variety of colorful fruits and vegetables into your diet to provide essential vitamins, minerals, antioxidants, and fiber. Aim for at least five servings per day to support overall health and fetal development.
- **Whole Grains:** Choose whole grain options such as brown rice, quinoa, whole wheat bread, and oatmeal for

their fiber, vitamins, and minerals. Whole grains provide sustained energy and help regulate blood sugar levels.

- **Lean Protein Sources:** Include lean sources of protein in your diet, such as poultry, fish, eggs, tofu, legumes, and nuts. Protein is essential for fetal growth and development, as well as maternal tissue repair and hormone production.
- **Dairy or Dairy Alternatives:** Consume dairy products or fortified dairy alternatives such as almond milk or soy milk to ensure an adequate intake of calcium and vitamin D. Choose low-fat or fat-free options to reduce saturated fat intake.
- **Healthy Fats:** Incorporate sources of healthy fats into your diet, such as avocados, nuts, seeds, and olive oil. These fats provide essential fatty acids and support fetal brain and eye development.

Foods to Limit or Avoid During Pregnancy

- **High-Mercury Fish:** Limit consumption of certain types of fish that are high in mercury, such as shark, swordfish, king mackerel, and tilefish. These fish can accumulate high levels of mercury, which can be harmful to the developing nervous system of the fetus.
- **Raw or Undercooked Seafood:** Avoid raw or undercooked seafood, including

sushi, sashimi, and shellfish, as they may contain harmful bacteria or parasites that can cause foodborne illness.

- **Unpasteurized Dairy Products:** Avoid unpasteurized dairy products such as raw milk, soft cheeses, and certain types of yogurt, as they may contain harmful bacteria such as Listeria monocytogenes, which can cause miscarriage, stillbirth, or other serious health complications.
- **Deli Meats and Refrigerated Pâtés:** Limit consumption of deli meats, hot dogs, and refrigerated pâtés, as they may be contaminated with Listeria monocytogenes. If consuming these foods, heat them until steaming hot to kill any potential bacteria.
- **Excessive Caffeine:** Limit caffeine intake to no more than 200 milligrams per day, as excessive caffeine consumption has been associated with an increased risk of miscarriage and low birth weight. Be mindful of hidden sources of caffeine, such as coffee, tea, soda, and chocolate.

Nutritional Benefits and Risks

Provide information on the nutritional benefits of the foods to include during pregnancy, as well as the potential risks associated with those to limit or avoid. Explain how certain nutrients support fetal development and maternal health, while also highlighting the importance of minimizing exposure to harmful substances that may pose risks to pregnancy outcomes.

Conclusion: Making informed food choices is essential for promoting a healthy pregnancy and supporting the health and development of both the mother and the baby. By including nutrient-rich foods in your diet and avoiding potentially harmful substances, you can optimize pregnancy outcomes and lay the foundation for a lifetime of good health. Consult with a healthcare provider or registered dietitian for personalized nutrition advice and guidance throughout pregnancy.

Chapter 4: Managing Common Pregnancy Symptoms

Introduction to Common Pregnancy Symptoms

Pregnancy is a time of significant physical and hormonal changes, which can often lead to discomfort and unpleasant symptoms for many women. In this chapter, we will address some of the most common pregnancy symptoms such as nausea, heartburn, and constipation, and provide dietary strategies for managing these symptoms.

Nausea and Morning Sickness

- **Ginger:** Incorporate ginger into your diet in various forms, such as ginger tea, ginger ale, or ginger candies. Ginger has natural anti-nausea properties and may help alleviate symptoms of morning sickness.
- **Frequent, Small Meals:** Eat frequent, small meals throughout the day to help prevent nausea and maintain stable blood sugar levels. Avoiding large meals and opting for lighter, more frequent snacks can help minimize feelings of nausea.
- **High-Carbohydrate Snacks:** Choose high-carbohydrate snacks such as crackers, toast, or dry cereal, which are often better tolerated during periods of nausea. These bland, easy-to-digest foods may help settle the stomach and alleviate symptoms.
- **Hydration:** Drink plenty of fluids throughout the day to stay hydrated, but avoid drinking large amounts of fluids with meals, as this can contribute to feelings of fullness and exacerbate nausea.

Heartburn

- **Smaller, More Frequent Meals:** Opt for smaller, more frequent meals to help prevent heartburn and reduce pressure on the stomach. Eating large meals can increase stomach acid production and exacerbate symptoms of heartburn.
- **Avoid Trigger Foods:** Identify and avoid foods that tend to trigger heartburn symptoms, such as spicy, greasy, or acidic foods, caffeine, and chocolate. Instead, focus on eating milder, less irritating foods that are easier on the digestive system.
- **Eat Slowly and Chew Thoroughly:** Take your time when eating, and chew your food slowly and thoroughly to aid digestion and prevent reflux. Eating too quickly can lead to swallowing air, which can worsen symptoms of heartburn.
- **Stay Upright After Eating:** Remain upright for at least 30 minutes after eating to help prevent stomach acid from refluxing into the esophagus. Avoid lying down or reclining immediately after meals, as this can exacerbate symptoms of heartburn.

Constipation

- **Fiber-Rich Foods:** Incorporate plenty of fiber-rich foods into your diet, such as fruits, vegetables, whole grains, legumes, and nuts. Fiber helps soften stools and promote regular bowel movements, reducing the risk of constipation.

- **Stay Hydrated:** Drink plenty of water throughout the day to stay hydrated and support healthy digestion. Adequate hydration helps soften stools and make them easier to pass, preventing constipation.
- **Physical Activity:** Engage in regular physical activity, such as walking, swimming, or prenatal yoga, to help stimulate bowel movements and promote regularity. Physical activity can also help alleviate symptoms of constipation and improve overall well-being during pregnancy.
- **Prunes and Prune Juice:** Prunes and prune juice are natural laxatives that can help relieve constipation. Incorporate prunes into your diet or drink prune juice to help soften stools and promote bowel regularity.

Nutritional Considerations

Provide information on the nutritional considerations associated with managing common pregnancy symptoms, such as ensuring adequate intake of essential nutrients despite dietary modifications made to alleviate discomfort. Emphasize the importance of maintaining a balanced diet and consulting with a healthcare provider or registered dietitian for personalized nutrition advice and guidance.

Conclusion: Managing common pregnancy symptoms such as nausea, heartburn, and constipation can be challenging, but dietary strategies can help alleviate discomfort and promote overall well-being during pregnancy. By making simple modifications to your diet and lifestyle, you can effectively manage these symptoms and enjoy a more comfortable and enjoyable pregnancy experience. Consult with a healthcare provider or registered dietitian for personalized recommendations tailored to your individual needs and preferences.

Chapter 5: Weight Gain Guidelines During Pregnancy

Introduction to Healthy Weight Gain

Achieving appropriate weight gain during pregnancy is essential for the health and well-being of both the mother and the baby. In this chapter, we will discuss healthy weight gain guidelines during pregnancy and provide guidance on how to achieve it through diet and exercise.

Importance of Healthy Weight Gain

- **Supports Fetal Growth and Development:** Adequate weight gain during pregnancy provides essential nutrients and energy for the growing fetus, supporting healthy growth and development.
- **Reduces Risk of Pregnancy Complications:** Achieving appropriate weight gain can help reduce the risk of pregnancy complications such as preterm birth, low birth weight, and gestational diabetes.
- **Promotes Maternal Health:** Maintaining a healthy weight during pregnancy can reduce the risk of maternal health issues such as preeclampsia, cesarean delivery, and postpartum weight retention.

Weight Gain Recommendations

- **Based on Pre-Pregnancy Body Mass Index (BMI):** Weight gain recommendations during pregnancy are based on a woman's pre-pregnancy BMI category. These guidelines help ensure appropriate weight gain for optimal pregnancy outcomes.
- **General Guidelines:** On average, women with a healthy pre-pregnancy BMI (18.5-24.9) are advised to gain between 25-35 pounds during pregnancy. Underweight women (BMI <18.5) may need to gain more, while

overweight and obese women (BMI ≥25) may need to gain less.

- **First Trimester:** During the first trimester, weight gain is typically minimal, with most women gaining 1-5 pounds. Nausea and vomiting may affect appetite and contribute to slower weight gain during this time.
- **Second and Third Trimesters:** Weight gain tends to accelerate during the second and third trimesters, with most women gaining approximately 1 pound per week. Focus on gradual, steady weight gain to support fetal growth and maternal health.

Achieving Healthy Weight Gain Through Diet

- **Balanced Diet:** Focus on consuming a balanced diet that includes a variety of nutrient-rich foods from all food groups. Emphasize fruits, vegetables, whole grains, lean proteins, and healthy fats to meet increased nutritional needs during pregnancy.
- **Portion Control:** Practice portion control to avoid overeating and excessive weight gain. Pay attention to hunger and fullness cues, and aim to eat until satisfied rather than overly full.
- **Nutrient-Dense Foods:** Choose nutrient-dense foods that provide essential vitamins, minerals, and other nutrients without excess calories. Opt

for whole foods over processed foods and limit intake of sugary snacks and beverages.
- **Regular Meals and Snacks:** Eat regular meals and snacks throughout the day to maintain stable blood sugar levels and prevent excessive hunger, which can lead to overeating.

Achieving Healthy Weight Gain Through Exercise

- **Safe Exercises:** Engage in regular, moderate-intensity exercise that is safe for pregnancy, such as walking, swimming, prenatal yoga, or low-impact aerobics. Exercise can help control weight gain, improve mood, and reduce the risk of pregnancy complications.
- **Consult with Healthcare Provider:** Consult with your healthcare provider before starting or continuing any exercise routine during pregnancy. Your provider can offer personalized recommendations based on your individual health status and pregnancy.
- **Listen to Your Body:** Pay attention to how your body feels during exercise and adjust intensity or duration as needed. Avoid activities that involve high risk of falling or abdominal trauma, and stop exercising if you experience any discomfort, pain, or unusual symptoms.

Conclusion: Achieving healthy weight gain during pregnancy is essential for supporting fetal growth and development, reducing the risk of pregnancy complications, and promoting maternal health. By following weight gain guidelines, adopting a balanced diet, and engaging in safe exercise, women can optimize pregnancy outcomes and lay the foundation for a healthy start for their babies. Consult with a healthcare provider or registered dietitian for personalized recommendations tailored to your individual needs and circumstances.

Chapter 6: Special Considerations During Pregnancy

Introduction to Special Dietary Concerns

Pregnancy brings about unique dietary considerations, particularly for women with specific dietary preferences, food allergies or intolerances, and cultural or religious dietary practices. In this chapter, we will address these special considerations and provide guidance for navigating them during pregnancy.

Vegetarian or Vegan Diets

- **Nutritional Considerations:** Vegetarian and vegan diets can provide all the nutrients needed during pregnancy with careful planning. Emphasize the importance of consuming a variety of plant-based foods to ensure adequate intake of protein, iron, calcium, vitamin D, omega-3 fatty acids, and other essential nutrients.
- **Protein Sources:** Include a variety of plant-based protein sources such as beans, lentils, tofu, tempeh, nuts, seeds, and whole grains in your diet. Combining different protein sources throughout the day can help ensure you're getting all the essential amino acids.
- **Iron-Rich Foods:** Incorporate iron-rich plant foods such as dark leafy greens, legumes, fortified cereals, and dried fruits into your meals to support iron absorption and prevent iron deficiency anemia.
- **Supplementation:** Consider taking a prenatal vitamin and mineral supplement to ensure you're meeting your increased nutritional needs during pregnancy. Some vegetarian and vegan women may need additional supplementation for nutrients such as vitamin B12, iron, and omega-3 fatty acids.

Food Allergies or Intolerances

- **Identifying Allergens:** If you have a known food allergy or intolerance, carefully read food labels and avoid foods that contain allergens or trigger symptoms. Common allergens include peanuts, tree nuts, dairy, eggs, soy, wheat, fish, and shellfish.
- **Substitution Options:** Identify alternative foods that can be safely substituted for allergenic ingredients in recipes. Explore allergy-friendly cooking and baking techniques, and consider using ingredient substitutions or alternative cooking methods to accommodate dietary restrictions.
- **Consult with Healthcare Provider:** Consult with your healthcare provider or a registered dietitian if you have food allergies or intolerances to ensure you're meeting your nutritional needs during pregnancy. They can provide personalized recommendations and guidance for managing dietary restrictions.

Cultural or Religious Dietary Practices

- **Respect Cultural and Religious Beliefs:** Respect cultural and religious dietary practices that may influence food choices and meal preparation during pregnancy. Understand the significance of certain foods or dietary restrictions and work to accommodate these preferences while ensuring optimal nutrition.

- **Flexibility and Adaptation:** Find ways to adapt traditional recipes or meals to meet your nutritional needs during pregnancy. Explore alternative ingredients or cooking methods that align with cultural or religious dietary guidelines while providing essential nutrients for you and your baby.
- **Seek Guidance if Needed:** If you have questions or concerns about how to maintain cultural or religious dietary practices during pregnancy, seek guidance from a healthcare provider or registered dietitian. They can offer support and advice for balancing cultural and religious beliefs with nutritional requirements during this important time.

Conclusion

Navigating special dietary concerns during pregnancy requires careful consideration and planning to ensure optimal nutrition for both the mother and the baby. By addressing specific dietary preferences, food allergies or intolerances, and cultural or religious dietary practices, pregnant women can maintain a healthy diet that supports their individual needs and beliefs. Consult with a healthcare provider or registered dietitian for personalized guidance and recommendations tailored to your unique circumstances.

Chapter 7: Supplements During Pregnancy

Introduction to Supplements

Supplements play a crucial role in supporting maternal and fetal health during pregnancy by providing essential vitamins, minerals, and other nutrients that may be challenging to obtain through diet alone. In this chapter, we will explain the role of prenatal vitamins and other supplements during pregnancy, including when and how to take them effectively.

Prenatal Vitamins

- **Purpose:** Prenatal vitamins are specially formulated multivitamin and mineral supplements designed to support the increased nutritional needs of pregnant women. They help ensure adequate intake of essential nutrients that are vital for fetal growth and development.

- **Key Nutrients:** Prenatal vitamins typically contain key nutrients such as folic acid, iron, calcium, vitamin D, omega-3 fatty acids, and other vitamins and minerals important for pregnancy.
- **When to Start:** It's recommended to start taking prenatal vitamins ideally before conception or as soon as pregnancy is confirmed. Early supplementation helps support fetal development during the critical early stages of pregnancy.
- **How to Take:** Take prenatal vitamins as directed by your healthcare provider, usually once daily with a meal to enhance absorption and minimize gastrointestinal discomfort. Avoid taking prenatal vitamins on an empty stomach, as this may increase the risk of nausea.
- **Choosing a Supplement:** Look for prenatal vitamins that contain adequate amounts of key nutrients, are free from unnecessary additives or fillers, and have been tested for quality and safety by a reputable third-party organization.

Folic Acid

- **Importance:** Folic acid, a B vitamin, is crucial for preventing neural tube defects (such as spina bifida) in the developing fetus. Adequate folic acid intake before conception and during early pregnancy is essential for reducing the risk of these birth defects.

- **Recommended Intake:** The recommended daily intake of folic acid for pregnant women is 600 micrograms (mcg) per day. Some women may require higher doses under the guidance of their healthcare provider, especially those with a history of neural tube defects or certain medical conditions.
- **Sources:** In addition to prenatal vitamins, folic acid can be obtained from fortified foods such as breakfast cereals, leafy green vegetables, legumes, and citrus fruits.

Iron

- **Importance:** Iron is essential for producing hemoglobin, the protein in red blood cells that carries oxygen to tissues and organs. During pregnancy, iron requirements increase to support the expansion of maternal blood volume and the development of the placenta and fetus.
- **Recommended Intake:** The recommended daily intake of iron for pregnant women is 27 milligrams (mg) per day. Iron deficiency during pregnancy can lead to anemia, fatigue, and increased risk of preterm birth and low birth weight.

- **Sources:** In addition to prenatal vitamins, iron can be obtained from iron-rich foods such as lean meats, poultry, fish, fortified cereals, legumes, and leafy green vegetables.

Calcium and Vitamin D

- **Importance:** Calcium and vitamin D are essential for supporting bone health and skeletal development in both the mother and the baby. Adequate intake of these nutrients during pregnancy helps prevent maternal bone loss and reduces the risk of conditions such as preeclampsia and preterm birth.
- **Recommended Intake:** The recommended daily intake of calcium for pregnant women is 1,000 to 1,300 milligrams (mg) per day, while the recommended intake of vitamin D is 600 international units (IU) per day.
- **Sources:** In addition to prenatal vitamins, calcium and vitamin D can be obtained from dairy products, fortified dairy alternatives, leafy green vegetables, canned fish with edible bones, and sunlight exposure.

Omega-3 Fatty Acids

- **Importance:** Omega-3 fatty acids, particularly DHA, play a crucial role in fetal brain and eye development. Adequate intake of omega-3 fatty acids during pregnancy is associated with improved cognitive development and reduced risk of certain pregnancy complications.

- **Recommended Intake:** The recommended intake of omega-3 fatty acids, specifically DHA, during pregnancy is at least 200 to 300 milligrams (mg) per day.
- **Sources:** In addition to prenatal vitamins, omega-3 fatty acids can be obtained from fatty fish such as salmon, mackerel, and sardines, as well as fish oil supplements.

Other Considerations

- **Consult with Healthcare Provider:** Before starting any supplementation regimen during pregnancy, consult with your healthcare provider or a registered dietitian to determine your individual nutrient needs and ensure that supplements are safe and appropriate for you.
- **Quality and Safety:** Choose prenatal vitamins and other supplements from reputable brands that have been tested for quality, purity, and safety by a third-party organization such as the United States Pharmacopeia (USP) or ConsumerLab.

- **Potential Risks:** While supplements can be beneficial, taking excessive amounts of certain vitamins and minerals can be harmful and may increase the risk of toxicity or adverse effects. Follow recommended dosages and avoid taking additional supplements without consulting your healthcare provider.

Conclusion:

Supplements, including prenatal vitamins and specific nutrients such as folic acid, iron, calcium, vitamin D, and omega-3 fatty acids, play a vital role in supporting maternal and fetal health during pregnancy. By following recommended guidelines for supplementation and consulting with healthcare providers as needed, pregnant women can ensure they're meeting their increased nutritional needs and optimizing pregnancy outcomes.

Chapter 8: Hydration During Pregnancy

Introduction to Hydration

Staying hydrated is essential for overall health, and it becomes even more crucial during pregnancy. In this chapter, we will emphasize the importance of staying hydrated during pregnancy and provide practical tips for increasing fluid intake to support maternal and fetal well-being.

Importance of Hydration During Pregnancy

- **Regulates Body Temperature:** Adequate hydration helps regulate body temperature, which is particularly important during pregnancy as the body's temperature may rise slightly due to increased metabolic activity.
- **Supports Nutrient Transport:** Water plays a crucial role in transporting nutrients to cells and removing waste products from the body. Maintaining proper hydration ensures efficient nutrient delivery to the developing fetus and supports maternal health.
- **Prevents Dehydration:** Dehydration during pregnancy can lead to various complications, including urinary tract infections, constipation, preterm labor, and low amniotic fluid levels. Staying well-hydrated helps prevent these issues and supports optimal pregnancy outcomes.

Hydration Recommendations

- **Daily Fluid Intake:** Pregnant women should aim to consume approximately 8-10 cups (64-80 ounces) of fluid per day, in addition to fluids obtained from food and other beverages.
- **Thirst as a Guide:** Use thirst as a guide for fluid intake, but also be mindful of other factors that may increase fluid needs, such as physical activity, hot weather, or certain medical conditions.
- **Urine Color:** Monitor urine color as an indicator of hydration status. Pale yellow urine generally indicates adequate hydration, while darker urine may suggest dehydration and the need to drink more fluids.

Tips for Increasing Fluid Intake

- **Drink Water Regularly:** Make water your primary beverage choice and drink it throughout the day. Keep a reusable water bottle with you to remind yourself to drink regularly.
- **Flavor Infusions:** Infuse water with natural flavors such as citrus slices, berries, cucumber, or mint to add variety and encourage consumption.
- **Herbal Teas:** Enjoy herbal teas such as peppermint, chamomile, or ginger tea, which can provide hydration along with potential health benefits.
- **Fruit and Vegetable Juices:** Include fruit and vegetable juices as part of your

fluid intake, but be mindful of added sugars and limit consumption of sweetened beverages.

- **Hydrating Foods:** Consume foods with high water content, such as fruits (e.g., watermelon, oranges, grapes) and vegetables (e.g., cucumber, celery, lettuce), to increase fluid intake while also obtaining essential nutrients.
- **Soups and Broths:** Incorporate soups, broths, and hydrating stews into your meals, particularly during colder weather, to boost fluid intake and add variety to your diet.

Special Considerations

- **Nausea and Vomiting:** If experiencing nausea and vomiting, focus on consuming small, frequent sips of water throughout the day to stay hydrated. Ginger tea or ginger-infused water may also help alleviate nausea.
- **Caffeine Intake:** Limit consumption of caffeinated beverages such as coffee, tea, and soda, as excessive caffeine intake can have diuretic effects and contribute to dehydration.
- **Alcohol Avoidance:** Avoid alcohol entirely during pregnancy, as it can harm the developing fetus and increase the risk of birth defects and other adverse outcomes.

Conclusion

Staying hydrated is essential for supporting maternal health and fetal development during pregnancy. By following hydration recommendations and implementing practical tips for increasing fluid intake, pregnant women can ensure they're meeting their increased fluid needs and promoting optimal pregnancy outcomes. Listen to your body's thirst cues, monitor urine color, and prioritize hydration as an integral part of your prenatal care routine.

Chapter 9: Postpartum Nutrition

Introduction to Postpartum Nutrition

The postpartum period is a critical time for maternal recovery and the establishment of breastfeeding, making proper nutrition essential for both maternal health and the well-being of the newborn. In this chapter, we will delve into the importance of postpartum nutrition, including recommendations for breastfeeding mothers and strategies for supporting recovery from childbirth.

Nutritional Needs During the Postpartum Period

- **Increased Energy Needs:** The postpartum period is characterized by increased energy demands due to breastfeeding, tissue repair, and hormonal fluctuations. Breastfeeding mothers require additional calories to support milk production and sustain their own energy levels.
- **Nutrient Replenishment:** Nutrients such as iron, calcium, vitamin D, and omega-3 fatty acids are particularly important during the postpartum period for replenishing maternal stores and supporting overall health and well-being.
- **Hydration:** Adequate hydration is crucial during the postpartum period, especially for breastfeeding mothers, as fluid needs increase to support milk production and prevent dehydration.

Nutrition Recommendations for Breastfeeding Mothers

- **Caloric Intake:** Breastfeeding mothers should aim to consume an additional 300-500 calories per day above their pre-pregnancy energy needs to support milk production and maternal health.
- **Nutrient-Dense Foods:** Focus on consuming nutrient-dense foods such as

fruits, vegetables, whole grains, lean proteins, and healthy fats to meet increased nutritional needs while providing optimal nourishment for the baby.

- **Omega-3 Fatty Acids:** Include sources of omega-3 fatty acids in your diet, such as fatty fish (e.g., salmon, sardines), flaxseeds, chia seeds, and walnuts, to support brain development and immune function in both the mother and the baby.
- **Hydration:** Drink plenty of fluids throughout the day, with water being the best choice. Aim to drink to thirst and pay attention to urine color as a guide for hydration status.

Recovery from Childbirth

- **Nutrient-Rich Foods:** Consume nutrient-rich foods that support tissue repair and replenish maternal stores of vitamins and minerals. Focus on incorporating foods high in iron, calcium, vitamin C, and protein to support healing and recovery.
- **Iron-Rich Foods:** Include iron-rich foods such as lean meats, poultry, fish, fortified cereals, legumes, and leafy green vegetables to replenish iron stores depleted during childbirth and prevent postpartum anemia.

- **Calcium Sources:** Incorporate calcium-rich foods such as dairy products, fortified dairy alternatives, leafy green vegetables, and calcium-fortified foods into your diet to support bone health and prevent calcium depletion.
- **Protein Intake:** Ensure an adequate intake of protein from sources such as lean meats, poultry, fish, eggs, dairy products, legumes, nuts, and seeds to support tissue repair and muscle recovery.

Special Considerations

- **Dietary Restrictions:** If you have any dietary restrictions or food allergies, work with a healthcare provider or registered dietitian to ensure you're meeting your nutritional needs while accommodating your dietary preferences or restrictions.
- **Supplementation:** Consider continuing to take a prenatal vitamin or specific supplements, such as iron or omega-3 fatty acids, during the postpartum period to support ongoing nutritional needs.
- **Seeking Support:** Reach out to a lactation consultant, healthcare provider, or support group for guidance and support with breastfeeding, nutrition, and postpartum recovery. Don't hesitate to ask for help if you're struggling or

have questions about your diet or breastfeeding journey.

Conclusion

Proper nutrition during the postpartum period is essential for maternal recovery, breastfeeding success, and overall well-being. By focusing on nutrient-dense foods, staying hydrated, and seeking support as needed, mothers can support their own health and provide optimal nourishment for their babies during this important time. Listen to your body's cues, prioritize self-care, and remember that nourishing yourself is key to caring for your newborn.

Chapter 10: Mindful Eating and Self-Care During Pregnancy

Introduction to Mindful Eating and Self-Care

Mindful eating and self-care practices are essential components of a healthy pregnancy, supporting both physical and emotional well-being for both the mother and the baby. In this chapter, we will explore the importance of mindfulness around eating and self-care practices during pregnancy, providing practical strategies for incorporating these principles into daily life.

Mindful Eating During Pregnancy

- **Awareness of Hunger and Fullness:** Practice tuning into your body's hunger and fullness cues, eating when hungry, and stopping when satisfied. Avoid eating out of boredom, stress, or other emotional triggers.
- **Savoring Food:** Take time to savor and appreciate each bite of food, paying attention to flavors, textures, and sensations. Eating slowly and mindfully can enhance the enjoyment of meals and promote satisfaction.
- **Emotional Eating:** Be mindful of emotional eating patterns and find alternative ways to cope with emotions such as stress, anxiety, or boredom. Engage in activities such as deep breathing, meditation, or gentle exercise to manage emotions without turning to food.
- **Connection to Food:** Cultivate a deeper connection to the food you eat by learning about where it comes from, how it's grown or produced, and the nutritional benefits it provides. Choose whole, minimally processed foods

whenever possible to nourish your body and support optimal health.

Self-Care Practices During Pregnancy

- **Physical Activity:** Engage in regular physical activity that is safe and appropriate for pregnancy, such as walking, swimming, prenatal yoga, or gentle stretching. Exercise not only supports physical health but also boosts mood and reduces stress.
- **Rest and Relaxation:** Prioritize rest and relaxation by incorporating relaxation techniques such as deep breathing, meditation, or progressive muscle relaxation into your daily routine. Adequate rest is essential for replenishing energy levels and supporting overall well-being.
- **Pampering Rituals:** Treat yourself to regular self-care rituals such as warm baths, prenatal massages, or soothing skincare routines. Taking time to pamper yourself can help alleviate stress, promote relaxation, and enhance feelings of self-love and appreciation.
- **Connection with Others:** Seek social support and connection with loved ones, friends, or support groups during pregnancy. Share your thoughts, feelings, and experiences with others who can provide empathy, encouragement, and understanding.

- **Mind-Body Practices:** Explore mind-body practices such as mindfulness meditation, guided imagery, or prenatal mindfulness classes to cultivate a sense of calm and presence during pregnancy. These practices can help reduce anxiety, enhance resilience, and promote emotional well-being.

Integrating Mindful Eating and Self-Care

- **Mealtime Rituals:** Create a supportive environment for mindful eating by establishing mealtime rituals such as setting the table with care, lighting candles, or playing soothing music. Engage in conversation and connection with family members or loved ones during meals.

Conclusion

Mindful eating and self-care practices are powerful tools for promoting physical and emotional well-being during pregnancy. By incorporating mindfulness into eating habits and prioritizing self-care practices, pregnant women can nourish their bodies, minds, and spirits, laying the foundation for a healthy and fulfilling pregnancy journey. Remember to listen to your body's needs, honor your emotions, and approach each day with kindness and compassion towards yourself.

Chapter 11: Consulting Healthcare Professionals During Pregnancy

Introduction to Consulting Healthcare Professionals

Consulting healthcare professionals, including obstetricians, midwives, and registered dietitians, is essential for ensuring optimal maternal and fetal health during pregnancy. In this chapter, we will stress the importance of seeking personalized nutrition advice and guidance from healthcare providers throughout pregnancy.

Role of Obstetricians and Midwives

- **Prenatal Care:** Obstetricians and midwives play a crucial role in providing prenatal care and monitoring the progress of pregnancy. Regular prenatal visits allow healthcare providers to assess maternal and fetal health, address any concerns or complications, and provide guidance for a healthy pregnancy.

- **Medical Monitoring:** Obstetricians and midwives monitor key indicators such as maternal weight gain, blood pressure, fetal growth, and fetal heart rate to ensure that both mother and baby are progressing as expected. They can also perform routine prenatal screenings and diagnostic tests to detect and manage any potential issues.
- **Educational Support:** Healthcare providers offer educational support and resources to help pregnant women understand their nutritional needs, manage pregnancy symptoms, and prepare for childbirth and parenthood. They can address questions and concerns related to diet, exercise, weight gain, and overall well-being.

Role of Registered Dietitians

- **Nutritional Assessment:** Registered dietitians (RDs) are trained experts in nutrition who can conduct a comprehensive assessment of a pregnant woman's dietary intake, nutritional status, and health history. They can identify any nutrient deficiencies or imbalances and provide personalized recommendations to optimize maternal and fetal nutrition.
- **Individualized Counseling:** RDs offer individualized nutrition counseling and guidance tailored to each woman's

specific needs, preferences, and health goals. They can help pregnant women navigate dietary restrictions, food allergies or intolerances, cultural or religious dietary practices, and other unique considerations.

- **Nutrition Education:** RDs provide evidence-based nutrition education on topics such as prenatal vitamins, nutrient-rich foods, hydration, weight management, and special dietary considerations during pregnancy. They empower women to make informed choices about their diet and lifestyle to support a healthy pregnancy.
- **Collaborative Care:** RDs work collaboratively with obstetricians, midwives, and other members of the healthcare team to ensure coordinated and comprehensive care for pregnant women. They communicate regularly with other healthcare providers to share information, coordinate interventions, and optimize outcomes for mother and baby.

Importance of Collaboration

- **Holistic Approach:** Collaborative care between obstetricians, midwives, and registered dietitians ensures a holistic approach to pregnancy care that addresses both medical and nutritional needs. This multidisciplinary approach considers the interconnectedness of physical, emotional, and social factors that influence maternal and fetal health.

- **Personalized Care:** By consulting with healthcare professionals, pregnant women can receive personalized nutrition advice and guidance tailored to their individual needs and circumstances. This personalized approach helps optimize maternal nutrition, support fetal development, and promote overall well-being during pregnancy.
- **Early Intervention:** Consulting with healthcare professionals early in pregnancy allows for early detection and management of any nutritional deficiencies, pregnancy complications, or other health concerns. Early intervention can help prevent or mitigate potential risks and improve pregnancy outcomes.
- **Continuity of Care:** Establishing a relationship with healthcare providers early in pregnancy promotes continuity of care throughout the prenatal period, childbirth, and postpartum recovery. Continuity of care ensures that women receive consistent support, monitoring, and guidance from trusted healthcare professionals at every stage of pregnancy.

Conclusion

Consulting with healthcare professionals, including obstetricians, midwives, and registered dietitians, is paramount for ensuring a healthy and successful pregnancy journey. By seeking personalized nutrition advice and guidance from qualified experts, pregnant women can access the support, resources, and education they need to optimize their health and well-being for themselves and their babies. Remember to prioritize regular prenatal care, open communication with healthcare providers, and collaboration among members of the healthcare team to promote the best possible outcomes for mother and baby.

Chapter 12: Meal Planning and Recipes for Pregnancy

Introduction to Meal Planning

Meal planning is an essential aspect of maintaining a healthy diet during pregnancy, ensuring that pregnant women meet their increased nutritional needs while enjoying delicious and satisfying meals. In this chapter, we will provide sample meal plans and recipes tailored to meet the nutritional needs of pregnant women, including options for different dietary preferences and restrictions.

Nutritional Considerations During Pregnancy

- **Macronutrients:** A balanced diet for pregnancy should include adequate amounts of carbohydrates, proteins, and fats to support maternal health and fetal development. Aim for a variety of nutrient-rich sources of each macronutrient to ensure comprehensive nutrition.
- **Micronutrients:** Pay attention to key micronutrients such as folic acid, iron, calcium, vitamin D, and omega-3 fatty acids, which are particularly important during pregnancy. Incorporate foods rich in these nutrients into your meals to support maternal and fetal health.
- **Hydration:** Stay hydrated by drinking plenty of fluids throughout the day, with water being the best choice. Aim to consume at least 8-10 cups of fluid per day, in addition to fluids obtained from food and other beverages.

Sample Meal Plans

Below are sample meal plans for pregnant women, designed to provide balanced nutrition and meet increased energy and nutrient needs during pregnancy.

Sample Meal Plan 1: Balanced Diet

- Breakfast: Greek yogurt with mixed berries and almonds
- Snack: Apple slices with peanut butter
- Lunch: Quinoa salad with mixed vegetables, chickpeas, and feta cheese
- Snack: Carrot sticks with hummus
- Dinner: Grilled salmon with roasted sweet potatoes and steamed broccoli

Sample Meal Plan 2: Vegetarian Diet

- Breakfast: Spinach and feta omelet with whole wheat toast
- Snack: Greek yogurt with granola and sliced banana
- Lunch: Lentil soup with whole grain roll and mixed green salad
- Snack: Trail mix with dried fruits and nuts
- Dinner: Tofu stir-fry with brown rice and mixed vegetables

Sample Meal Plan 3: Vegan Diet

- Breakfast: Overnight oats with almond milk, chia seeds, and mixed berries

- Snack: Homemade energy balls made with dates, nuts, and cocoa powder
- Lunch: Chickpea salad wrap with avocado, lettuce, and tomato
- Snack: Sliced cucumber with tahini
- Dinner: Lentil curry with quinoa and steamed spinach

Recipes

Below are recipes for nutritious and delicious meals that are suitable for pregnant women:

- **Quinoa Salad with Mixed Vegetables and Chickpeas**
  - Ingredients:
    - Cooked quinoa
    - Mixed vegetables (bell peppers, cucumbers, tomatoes, etc.)
    - Cooked chickpeas
    - Feta cheese (optional)
    - Olive oil
    - Lemon juice
    - Salt and pepper to taste
  - Instructions: Combine cooked quinoa, mixed vegetables, and chickpeas in a bowl. Drizzle with olive oil and lemon juice, then season with salt and pepper. Sprinkle with feta cheese if desired.

- **Tofu Stir-Fry with Brown Rice and Mixed Vegetables**
  - Ingredients:
    - Firm tofu, cubed
    - Mixed vegetables (bell peppers, broccoli, carrots, etc.)
    - Soy sauce
    - Garlic, minced
    - Ginger, grated
    - Brown rice, cooked
  - Instructions: In a skillet, stir-fry tofu cubes until golden brown. Add mixed vegetables, garlic, and ginger, and cook until vegetables are tender. Drizzle with soy sauce and serve over cooked brown rice.

- **Chickpea Salad Wrap with Avocado**
  - Ingredients:
    - Canned chickpeas, drained and rinsed
    - Mixed salad greens
    - Avocado, sliced
    - Whole grain wraps
    - Hummus
  - Instructions: Mash chickpeas with a fork and mix with hummus. Spread chickpea mixture onto whole grain wraps. Top with mixed salad greens and sliced avocado. Roll up

wraps and serve.

- **Salmon and Quinoa Bowl**
  - Ingredients:
    - Cooked quinoa
    - Grilled or baked salmon fillet
    - Steamed broccoli florets
    - Sliced avocado
    - Lemon wedges
    - Olive oil
    - Salt and pepper to taste
  - Instructions: Assemble cooked quinoa, grilled or baked salmon, steamed broccoli, and sliced avocado in a bowl. Drizzle with olive oil, squeeze fresh lemon juice over the top, and season with salt and pepper.

- **Vegetable Stir-Fry with Tofu**
  - Ingredients:
    - Firm tofu, cubed
    - Mixed vegetables (bell peppers, snap peas, carrots, etc.)
    - Soy sauce
    - Garlic, minced
    - Ginger, grated
    - Sesame oil
    - Cooked rice or noodles
  - Instructions: In a wok or skillet, stir-fry tofu cubes until lightly browned. Add mixed

vegetables, garlic, and ginger,
and cook until vegetables are
tender-crisp. Drizzle with soy
sauce and sesame oil, and
serve over cooked rice or
noodles.

- **Mango and Avocado Salad**
  - Ingredients:
    - Mixed salad greens
    - Ripe mango, diced
    - Avocado, diced
    - Red onion, thinly sliced
    - Cherry tomatoes,
      halved
    - Toasted pumpkin seeds
      (optional)
    - Balsamic vinaigrette
  - Instructions: Toss mixed salad
    greens with diced mango,
    avocado, sliced red onion, and
    halved cherry tomatoes.
    Sprinkle with toasted pumpkin
    seeds if desired and drizzle with
    balsamic vinaigrette before
    serving.

- **Black Bean and Sweet Potato Tacos**
  - Ingredients:
    - Corn tortillas
    - Canned black beans,
      drained and rinsed
    - Roasted sweet
      potatoes, diced

- Sliced avocado
- Salsa or pico de gallo
- Fresh cilantro leaves
- Lime wedges
    - Instructions: Warm corn tortillas and fill with black beans, roasted sweet potatoes, sliced avocado, and salsa or pico de gallo. Garnish with fresh cilantro leaves and serve with lime wedges for squeezing.

- **Greek Yogurt Parfait with Berries and Granola**
    - Ingredients:
        - Greek yogurt
        - Mixed berries (strawberries, blueberries, raspberries)
        - Granola
        - Honey or maple syrup (optional)
    - Instructions: Layer Greek yogurt, mixed berries, and granola in a glass or bowl to create a parfait. Drizzle with honey or maple syrup if desired for added sweetness.

- **Vegetable and Lentil Soup**
    - Ingredients:
        - 1 cup dried lentils
        - 4 cups vegetable broth

- 1 onion, diced
        - 2 carrots, diced
        - 2 celery stalks, diced
        - 2 cloves garlic, minced
        - 1 teaspoon dried thyme
        - 1 teaspoon dried oregano
        - Salt and pepper to taste
        - Fresh parsley, chopped (for garnish)
    - Instructions: In a large pot, combine lentils, vegetable broth, onion, carrots, celery, garlic, thyme, and oregano. Bring to a boil, then reduce heat and simmer for 20-25 minutes or until lentils are tender. Season with salt and pepper to taste. Serve hot, garnished with fresh parsley.

- **Sweet Potato and Black Bean Quesadillas**
- Ingredients:
    - 2 large sweet potatoes, peeled and diced
    - 1 can black beans, drained and rinsed
    - 1 teaspoon ground cumin
    - 1/2 teaspoon chili powder
    - 1/2 teaspoon paprika
    - Salt and pepper to taste
    - 4 large whole wheat tortillas

- - 1 cup shredded cheese (cheddar or Monterey Jack)
    - Olive oil (for cooking)
- Instructions: Steam or boil sweet potatoes until tender. In a large bowl, mash sweet potatoes with black beans, cumin, chili powder, paprika, salt, and pepper. Spread mixture evenly onto half of each tortilla, then sprinkle with shredded cheese. Fold tortillas in half to enclose filling. Heat olive oil in a skillet over medium heat, then cook quesadillas for 2-3 minutes on each side until golden brown and cheese is melted. Serve warm, sliced into wedges.

- **Pasta Primavera**
- Ingredients:
    - 8 ounces whole wheat pasta (such as penne or fusilli)
    - 2 tablespoons olive oil
    - 2 cloves garlic, minced
    - 1 onion, diced
    - 2 carrots, sliced
    - 1 bell pepper, diced
    - 1 zucchini, diced
    - 1 cup cherry tomatoes, halved
    - 1/2 cup vegetable broth
    - 1/4 cup grated Parmesan cheese
    - Fresh basil leaves, chopped (for garnish)
- Instructions: Cook pasta according to package instructions. Meanwhile, heat

olive oil in a large skillet over medium heat. Add garlic and onion, and cook until softened. Add carrots, bell pepper, and zucchini, and cook until tender-crisp. Stir in cherry tomatoes and vegetable broth, and simmer for 2-3 minutes. Toss cooked pasta with vegetable mixture, then sprinkle with grated Parmesan cheese and fresh basil before serving.

- **Fruit and Nut Salad with Honey-Lime Dressing**
- Ingredients:
    - Mixed salad greens
    - Sliced strawberries
    - Blueberries
    - Sliced almonds
    - Dried cranberries
    - Crumbled feta cheese
    - For the dressing:
        - 2 tablespoons olive oil
        - 1 tablespoon honey
        - 1 tablespoon lime juice
        - 1/2 teaspoon Dijon mustard
        - Salt and pepper to taste
- Instructions: In a small bowl, whisk together olive oil, honey, lime juice, Dijon mustard, salt, and pepper to make the dressing. In a large bowl, combine mixed salad greens, sliced strawberries, blueberries, sliced almonds, dried cranberries, and crumbled feta cheese.

Drizzle with honey-lime dressing just before serving.

- **Mediterranean Chickpea Salad**
- Ingredients:
    - 1 can chickpeas, drained and rinsed
    - 1 cucumber, diced
    - 1 bell pepper, diced
    - 1/4 red onion, thinly sliced
    - 1/2 cup cherry tomatoes, halved
    - 1/4 cup Kalamata olives, sliced
    - 2 tablespoons crumbled feta cheese
    - 2 tablespoons extra virgin olive oil
    - 1 tablespoon red wine vinegar
    - 1 teaspoon dried oregano
    - Salt and pepper to taste
- Instructions: In a large bowl, combine chickpeas, cucumber, bell pepper, red onion, cherry tomatoes, and Kalamata olives. In a small bowl, whisk together olive oil, red wine vinegar, dried oregano, salt, and pepper to make the dressing. Drizzle the dressing over the salad and toss to combine. Sprinkle with crumbled feta cheese before serving.

- **Asian-Inspired Tofu Stir-Fry**
- Ingredients:
    - 1 block firm tofu, pressed and cubed

- o 2 cups mixed vegetables (broccoli, bell peppers, snap peas, carrots, etc.)
  - o 2 cloves garlic, minced
  - o 1 tablespoon ginger, grated
  - o 2 tablespoons soy sauce
  - o 1 tablespoon hoisin sauce
  - o 1 tablespoon sesame oil
  - o Cooked rice or noodles for serving
  - o Sesame seeds and chopped green onions for garnish
- Instructions: In a wok or skillet, heat sesame oil over medium-high heat. Add cubed tofu and cook until golden brown on all sides. Remove tofu from the pan and set aside. In the same pan, add mixed vegetables, garlic, and ginger. Stir-fry until vegetables are tender-crisp. Return tofu to the pan and add soy sauce and hoisin sauce. Cook for an additional 1-2 minutes, stirring to coat everything evenly. Serve over cooked rice or noodles, garnished with sesame seeds and chopped green onions.

- **Caprese Stuffed Avocado**
- Ingredients:
  - o Ripe avocados, halved and pitted
  - o Cherry tomatoes, halved
  - o Fresh mozzarella cheese, diced
  - o Fresh basil leaves, torn
  - o Balsamic glaze for drizzling

- o   Salt and pepper to taste
- Instructions: Scoop out a little avocado flesh from each avocado half to create a hollow. Fill each avocado half with cherry tomatoes, fresh mozzarella cheese, and torn basil leaves. Drizzle with balsamic glaze and season with salt and pepper to taste. Serve immediately as a light and refreshing appetizer or snack.

- **Mango Coconut Chia Pudding**
- Ingredients:
  - o   1/4 cup chia seeds
  - o   1 cup coconut milk
  - o   1 ripe mango, diced
  - o   2 tablespoons shredded coconut (optional)
  - o   Honey or maple syrup for sweetness (optional)
- Instructions: In a bowl, whisk together chia seeds and coconut milk. Let it sit for 5 minutes, then whisk again to prevent clumps. Cover and refrigerate for at least 2 hours or overnight until thickened. Before serving, layer chia pudding with diced mango in serving glasses or jars. Optionally, sprinkle with shredded coconut and drizzle with honey or maple syrup for sweetness.

- **Roasted Vegetable Quinoa Bowl**
- Ingredients:
  - o   1 cup quinoa, rinsed

- o 2 cups mixed vegetables (such as bell peppers, zucchini, eggplant, and cherry tomatoes), chopped
  - o 2 tablespoons olive oil
  - o 2 cloves garlic, minced
  - o 1 teaspoon dried thyme
  - o Salt and pepper to taste
  - o Fresh parsley, chopped (for garnish)
- Instructions:
  - o Preheat the oven to 400°F (200°C).
  - o In a bowl, toss the mixed vegetables with olive oil, minced garlic, dried thyme, salt, and pepper until evenly coated.
  - o Spread the vegetables in a single layer on a baking sheet. Roast in the preheated oven for 20-25 minutes, or until tender and slightly caramelized.
  - o Meanwhile, cook the quinoa according to package instructions.
  - o To assemble the quinoa bowls, divide the cooked quinoa among serving bowls and top with the roasted vegetables. Garnish with chopped fresh parsley before serving.

- **Sesame Ginger Tofu Salad**
- Ingredients:

- o   1 block firm tofu, pressed and cubed
  - o   4 cups mixed salad greens
  - o   1 cucumber, sliced
  - o   1 carrot, julienned
  - o   1/4 cup sliced almonds
  - o   2 tablespoons sesame seeds
  - o   For the dressing:
    - ▪   2 tablespoons soy sauce
    - ▪   1 tablespoon rice vinegar
    - ▪   1 tablespoon sesame oil
    - ▪   1 tablespoon honey
    - ▪   1 teaspoon grated ginger
    - ▪   1 garlic clove, minced
- •   Instructions:
  - o   In a bowl, whisk together all the ingredients for the dressing until well combined.
  - o   In a skillet over medium heat, cook the cubed tofu until golden brown on all sides.
  - o   In a large salad bowl, combine the mixed salad greens, sliced cucumber, julienned carrot, sliced almonds, and sesame seeds.
  - o   Add the cooked tofu to the salad bowl and drizzle with the sesame ginger dressing. Toss gently to coat everything evenly

before serving.

- **Stuffed Bell Peppers with Quinoa and Black Beans**
- Ingredients:
    - 4 large bell peppers, halved and seeds removed
    - 1 cup cooked quinoa
    - 1 cup canned black beans, drained and rinsed
    - 1 cup corn kernels
    - 1/2 cup diced tomatoes
    - 1/4 cup chopped cilantro
    - 1 teaspoon ground cumin
    - 1 teaspoon chili powder
    - Salt and pepper to taste
    - Shredded cheese (optional, for topping)
- Instructions:
    - Preheat the oven to 375°F (190°C).
    - In a large bowl, combine the cooked quinoa, black beans, corn kernels, diced tomatoes, chopped cilantro, ground cumin, chili powder, salt, and pepper.
    - Spoon the quinoa mixture into each halved bell pepper until filled.
    - Place the stuffed bell peppers in a baking dish and cover with aluminum foil.

- Bake in the preheated oven for 25-30 minutes, or until the bell peppers are tender.
  - If desired, remove the foil, sprinkle shredded cheese on top of each stuffed bell pepper, and return to the oven for an additional 5 minutes until the cheese is melted and bubbly.
  - Serve hot as a nutritious and satisfying meal.

- **Banana Oatmeal Breakfast Muffins**
- Ingredients:
  - 2 ripe bananas, mashed
  - 2 cups rolled oats
  - 1/4 cup honey or maple syrup
  - 1/4 cup milk (dairy or plant-based)
  - 1 teaspoon vanilla extract
  - 1 teaspoon ground cinnamon
  - 1/2 teaspoon baking powder
  - Pinch of salt
  - Optional add-ins: chopped nuts, dried fruits, chocolate chips
- Instructions:
  - Preheat the oven to 350°F (175°C) and grease a muffin tin or line it with paper liners.
  - In a large mixing bowl, combine the mashed bananas, rolled oats, honey or maple syrup, milk, vanilla extract, ground

cinnamon, baking powder, and
salt. Mix until well combined.
- o   If using any optional add-ins,
  fold them into the batter.
- o   Divide the batter evenly among
  the prepared muffin cups, filling
  each about three-quarters full.
- o   Bake in the preheated oven for
  20-25 minutes, or until the
  muffins are golden brown and a
  toothpick inserted into the
  center comes out clean.
- o   Allow the muffins to cool in the
  pan for a few minutes before
  transferring them to a wire rack
  to cool completely.
- o   Enjoy the banana oatmeal
  breakfast muffins as a nutritious
  and portable breakfast option.

- **Lentil and Vegetable Curry**
- Ingredients:
  - o   1 cup dried lentils, rinsed
  - o   1 onion, diced
  - o   2 cloves garlic, minced
  - o   1 tablespoon curry powder
  - o   1 teaspoon ground turmeric
  - o   1 teaspoon ground cumin
  - o   1 can (14 oz) diced tomatoes
  - o   2 cups vegetable broth
  - o   2 cups mixed vegetables (such
    as carrots, bell peppers, and
    spinach), chopped
  - o   Salt and pepper to taste

- o Cooked rice or naan bread for serving
- Instructions:
    - o In a large pot, sauté the diced onion and minced garlic until softened.
    - o Add the curry powder, ground turmeric, and ground cumin to the pot, and cook for 1-2 minutes until fragrant.
    - o Stir in the diced tomatoes, vegetable broth, and rinsed lentils. Bring to a boil, then reduce heat and simmer for 20-25 minutes, or until the lentils are tender.
    - o Add the mixed vegetables to the pot and cook for an additional 5-10 minutes, until the vegetables are tender.
    - o Season the curry with salt and pepper to taste.
    - o Serve the lentil and vegetable curry over cooked rice or with naan bread for a hearty and flavorful meal.

- **Spinach and Feta Stuffed Chicken Breast**
- Ingredients:
    - o 4 boneless, skinless chicken breasts
    - o 2 cups fresh spinach leaves
    - o 1/2 cup crumbled feta cheese

- o 2 cloves garlic, minced
- o 1 tablespoon olive oil
- o Salt and pepper to taste
- Instructions:
  - o Preheat the oven to 375°F (190°C).
  - o Using a sharp knife, make a horizontal slit in each chicken breast to create a pocket.
  - o In a skillet, heat the olive oil over medium heat. Add the minced garlic and sauté until fragrant.
  - o Add the fresh spinach leaves to the skillet and cook until wilted. Remove from heat and stir in the crumbled feta cheese.
  - o Stuff each chicken breast with the spinach and feta mixture, then season with salt and pepper.
  - o Place the stuffed chicken breasts in a baking dish and bake in the preheated oven for 25-30 minutes, or until the chicken is cooked through and no longer pink in the center.
  - o Serve the spinach and feta stuffed chicken breasts with your favorite side dishes for a delicious and protein-packed meal.

- **Pumpkin and Chickpea Curry**

- Ingredients:
  - 1 tablespoon olive oil
  - 1 onion, diced
  - 2 cloves garlic, minced
  - 1 tablespoon curry powder
  - 1 teaspoon ground cumin
  - 1 teaspoon ground coriander
  - 1 can (14 oz) diced tomatoes
  - 1 can (14 oz) coconut milk
  - 1 can (14 oz) chickpeas, drained and rinsed
  - 1 cup pumpkin puree
  - Salt and pepper to taste
  - Fresh cilantro leaves, chopped (for garnish)
- Instructions:
  - In a large pot, heat the olive oil over medium heat. Add the diced onion and minced garlic, and sauté until softened.
  - Stir in the curry powder, ground cumin, and ground coriander, and cook for 1-2 minutes until fragrant.
  - Add the diced tomatoes (with their juices), coconut milk, drained chickpeas, and pumpkin puree to the pot. Stir to combine.
  - Bring the curry to a simmer, then reduce heat and cook for 15-20 minutes, stirring occasionally, until the flavors

are well combined and the pumpkin is cooked through.
  - Season the curry with salt and pepper to taste.
  - Serve the pumpkin and chickpea curry hot, garnished with chopped fresh cilantro leaves, and accompanied by rice or naan bread.

- **Mango Avocado Salsa**
- Ingredients:
  - 1 ripe mango, diced
  - 1 ripe avocado, diced
  - 1/4 cup red onion, finely chopped
  - 1/4 cup fresh cilantro leaves, chopped
  - 1 jalapeño pepper, seeded and minced
  - Juice of 1 lime
  - Salt and pepper to taste
- Instructions:
  - In a bowl, combine the diced mango, diced avocado, finely chopped red onion, chopped cilantro leaves, and minced jalapeño pepper.
  - Squeeze the juice of one lime over the salsa and gently toss to combine.
  - Season the salsa with salt and pepper to taste.

- o Serve the mango avocado salsa as a refreshing topping for grilled chicken, fish, tacos, or as a dip with tortilla chips.

- **Stuffed Bell Peppers with Quinoa and Black Beans**
- Ingredients:
    - o 4 large bell peppers, halved and seeds removed
    - o 1 cup cooked quinoa
    - o 1 cup canned black beans, drained and rinsed
    - o 1 cup corn kernels
    - o 1/2 cup diced tomatoes
    - o 1/4 cup chopped cilantro
    - o 1 teaspoon ground cumin
    - o 1 teaspoon chili powder
    - o Salt and pepper to taste
    - o Shredded cheese (optional, for topping)
- Instructions:
    - o Preheat the oven to 375°F (190°C).
    - o In a large bowl, mix together cooked quinoa, black beans, corn kernels, diced tomatoes, chopped cilantro, ground cumin, chili powder, salt, and pepper.
    - o Stuff each bell pepper half with the quinoa and black bean mixture.
    - o Place the stuffed bell peppers in a baking dish. If desired,

sprinkle shredded cheese on top.

- o Cover the baking dish with foil and bake for 25-30 minutes, or until the peppers are tender.
- o Remove the foil and bake for an additional 5 minutes to melt the cheese (if using).
- o Serve the stuffed bell peppers hot, garnished with extra cilantro if desired.

- **Coconut Curry Lentil Soup**
- Ingredients:
    - o 1 tablespoon coconut oil
    - o 1 onion, diced
    - o 2 cloves garlic, minced
    - o 1 tablespoon curry powder
    - o 1 teaspoon ground turmeric
    - o 1 teaspoon ground cumin
    - o 1 cup dried red lentils, rinsed
    - o 4 cups vegetable broth
    - o 1 can (14 oz) coconut milk
    - o 2 cups chopped kale or spinach
    - o Juice of 1 lime
    - o Salt and pepper to taste
    - o Fresh cilantro leaves, chopped (for garnish)
- Instructions:
    - o In a large pot, heat coconut oil over medium heat. Add diced onion and minced garlic, and sauté until softened.

- o   Stir in curry powder, ground turmeric, and ground cumin, and cook for 1-2 minutes until fragrant.
  - o   Add rinsed red lentils and vegetable broth to the pot. Bring to a boil, then reduce heat and simmer for 15-20 minutes, or until lentils are tender.
  - o   Stir in coconut milk and chopped kale or spinach, and simmer for an additional 5 minutes until the greens are wilted.
  - o   Remove from heat and stir in lime juice. Season with salt and pepper to taste.
  - o   Serve the coconut curry lentil soup hot, garnished with chopped fresh cilantro leaves.

- **Peanut Butter Banana Smoothie Bowl**
- Ingredients:
  - o   2 ripe bananas, frozen
  - o   1/4 cup creamy peanut butter
  - o   1/2 cup Greek yogurt
  - o   1/2 cup milk (dairy or plant-based)
  - o   2 tablespoons honey or maple syrup
  - o   Toppings: sliced bananas, granola, chopped nuts, shredded coconut
- Instructions:

- In a blender, combine frozen bananas, peanut butter, Greek yogurt, milk, and honey or maple syrup. Blend until smooth and creamy.
    - Pour the smoothie into bowls.
    - Top with sliced bananas, granola, chopped nuts, and shredded coconut, or any other desired toppings.
    - Serve the peanut butter banana smoothie bowls immediately for a nutritious and filling breakfast or snack.

- **Vegetarian Sushi Rolls**
- Ingredients:
    - Sushi rice
    - Nori seaweed sheets
    - Assorted fillings: thinly sliced cucumber, avocado, carrot matchsticks, bell pepper strips, tofu strips, etc.
    - Soy sauce, for dipping
    - Pickled ginger and wasabi, optional
- Instructions:
    - Cook sushi rice according to package instructions and let it cool to room temperature.
    - Place a nori seaweed sheet on a bamboo sushi mat or flat surface.

- o Spread a thin layer of sushi rice evenly over the nori sheet, leaving about an inch of space at the top.
  - o Arrange your desired fillings horizontally along the bottom edge of the rice.
  - o Roll the sushi tightly, using the bamboo mat to help shape and compress the roll.
  - o Wet the exposed edge of the nori sheet with water to seal the roll.
  - o Use a sharp knife to slice the sushi roll into individual pieces.
  - o Serve the vegetarian sushi rolls with soy sauce, pickled ginger, and wasabi on the side for dipping.

Conclusion

Meal planning and preparation are essential for maintaining a healthy diet during pregnancy, ensuring that pregnant women receive adequate nutrition to support maternal and fetal health. By following sample meal plans and incorporating nutritious recipes into their diets, pregnant women can enjoy delicious and satisfying meals that meet their increased energy and nutrient needs. Remember to consult with healthcare professionals for personalized nutrition advice and guidance tailored to your individual needs and preferences.

As we come to the end of this journey through nutrition during pregnancy, I hope these recipes and insights have provided you with valuable information and inspiration for nourishing yourself and your growing baby. Remember, pregnancy is a special time where the foods you eat play a crucial role in supporting both your health and the development of your little one.

As you continue on this remarkable journey, may you embrace the joy of preparing nutritious meals, savor the flavors of each bite, and cherish the moments shared around the table with loved ones. Wishing you a healthy and fulfilling pregnancy journey filled with abundant blessings and happiness.

Bon appétit and best wishes for a beautiful pregnancy and beyond!

www.ingramcontent.com/pod-product-compliance
Lightning Source LLC
Chambersburg PA
CBHW050821250726
48653CB00006B/2356